HOW-TO-GUIDE: PENICILLIN

How the first antibiotic transformed global healthcare

Dr. Bernard Johnson

Contents

CHAPTER ONE 4
- Introduction 4
- History and Discovery of Penicillin 9
- Development and Mass Production 14
- Types of Penicillins and Their Derivatives 29
- Bacterial Infections Treated with Penicillin 34

CHAPTER TWO 39
- Dosage and Administration 39
- Conditions to be Treated 43
- The Rise of Penicillin Resistance 46
- Mechanisms of Resistance 48
- Strategies to Overcome Resistance 53

CHAPTER THREE 57
- Penicillin Allergy and Side Effects 57
- Common Side Effects 59
- Serious Reactions and Anaphylaxis 61
- Penicillin in Modern Medicine 63
- Penicillin in Combination Therapy 68
- Alternatives to Penicillin 71

CHAPTER FOUR 76
- Antibiotic Resistance Being Tackled 76
- The Role of Penicillin in Emerging Infections 80
- The Ethics of Antibiotic Use 82
- Availability of Penicillin in Developing Countries 85
- Patent Issues and Generic Production 88
- Conclusion 90

Future Challenges and Innovations 93
THE END 100

CHAPTER ONE

Introduction

Penicillin is the first true antibiotic ever isolated by man, which has revolutionized medicine and saved countless lives. Before its discovery, bacterial infections were mostly terminal, with very few treatment options available. The introduction of penicillin in the 20th century heralded the antibiotic era, after which the face of infectious disease treatment changed beyond imagination.

This book speaks to multifarious dimensions of penicillin, reaching from the time of its discovery in history to the impact it had on modern medicine. We will attempt to delve into such things as its chemical structure, mechanism of action, clinical uses, and problems of resistance. We shall address the ethical considerations for antibiotic use and the future of penicillin if we face ever-increasing bacterial resistance.

History and Discovery of Penicillin

In 1928, the Scottish bacteriologist Alexander Fleming serendipitously made a discovery that changed medical history.

Having come back from vacation, Fleming noticed that one of his Petri dishes with Staphylococcus bacteria had been contaminated with mold that later turned out to be Penicillium notatum.

Surprisingly enough, the zone around the mold did not grow bacteria, which obviously proved that the mold secreted a substance inhibiting the growth of bacteria. The substance was penicillin.

When first discovered by Fleming, the substance was not received with a lot of enthusiasm because he could not isolate the active compound in large enough quantities. His findings, however, provided the basis for future research to be carried out which would later discover penicillin as a medicine.

Development and Mass Production

Mass production of penicillin greatly improved during World War II, as combatants realized that in order to conquer the various infections contracted during the war, they first needed to defeat the ones that were ravaging their own bodies. A young Rhodes scholar enrolled at

Oxford University by the name of Howard Florey, together with a biochemist also working at Oxford, Ernst Boris Chain, and Norman Heatley joined forces in developing a new, purer form of penicillin.

The work of Florey and Chain was focused on the purification of penicillin and testing it clinically, after which the discovery proved potent against bacterial infection. With this help from the U.S. and

British governments, production was scaled up industrially to enable the wide distribution of penicillin among Allied forces in the war.

In 1945, Alexander Fleming, Howard Florey,

and Ernst Boris Chain received the Nobel Prize in Physiology or Medicine for work on the discovery of penicillin. Penicillin did not remain confined to the battlefield, though; it moved quickly, after isolation, into civilian life and to this day is one of the most prescribed drugs for the treatment of a number of different types of bacterial infections.

The discovery and development of penicillin really did revolutionize medicine, reducing the mortality rates from most of the bacterial infections and discovering other antibiotics that followed after its invention.

Chemical Structure and Mechanism of Action

Penicillin is a beta-lactam antibiotic, identified by its four-membered beta-lactam ring. This ring is constituted by the part of the antibiotic that performs its bactericidal action. The overall structure for penicillin is a thiazolidine ring coupled to the beta-lactam ring with a variable substituent or side chain,

R, which determines the individual features and activity spectrum of the numerous penicillins.

How Penicillin Works

It achieves its antibacterial action by inhibiting the synthesis of bacterial cell walls, which is quite important in maintaining the structural integrity of the bacteria. The beta-lactam ring of penicillin binds to and inactivates enzymes known as penicillin-binding proteins involved in the final steps of the synthesis of the cell wall.

Due to this inhibition, cross-linking between the layers of peptidoglycan in the cell wall does not take place. In this type of action, penicillin is most effective against Gram-positive bacteria because it contains a thick layer of peptidoglycan. Eventually, the organism dies because of the lysis of the cell.

Types of Penicillins and Their Derivatives

During this time, there have been various types of penicillin and its derivatives developed in order to give coverage to an extended area of bacteria and to counter the resistance. These may be: Penicillin G: The oldest penicillin, most frequently applied against serious infections like syphilis, meningitis, and endocarditis.

Penicillin V: Phenoxymethylpenicillin is the oral form of penicillin; it is mainly indicated for milder infections caused by this antibiotic and includes tonsillopharyngitis, strep throat, and skin infections. Ampicillin and amoxicillin are broad-spectrum penicillins, acting against a wide variety of bacteria, frequently some Gram-negative.

Methicillin: Formulated against penicillin-resistant Staphylococcus aureus, now largely superseded by other antibiotics due to the development of resistance.

Bacterial Infections Treated with Penicillin

Penicillin is used to treat a number of bacterial infections, primarily caused by Gram-positive organisms. Some of the most common conditions treated using penicillin are as follows:

Streptococcal Infections: This antibiotic is applied in a variety of Streptococcus pyogenes infections like strep throat, scarlet fever, and rheumatic fever.

Syphilis: Syphilis is a sexually transmitted infection caused by the spirochete Treponema pallidum; its treatment of choice is penicillin G.

Meningitis: Treatment of bacterial meningitis may be done using penicillin in cases whose the infection is caused by Neisseria meningitidis and Streptococcus pneumoniae.

Endocarditis: Penicillin is indicated in the treatment of bacterial endocarditis, particularly caused by Streptococcus viridans or Enterococcus species.

CHAPTER TWO

Dosage and Administration

The dose and route of penicillin administration vary with the type and severity of infection and the patient's age, weight, and renal function.

Penicillin is given orally, intramuscularly, or intravenously.

Oral Penicillin V: is given in divided doses for mild

and medium-severity infections, as in strep throat or skin infections.

Intramuscular Penicillin G: it is used to treat syphilis and more serious infections. How often it is dosed depends on the stage of the particular disease being treated.

Intravenous Penicillin G: this route of administration is only warranted in severe infections like meningitis, endocarditis where high blood levels of this antibiotic are necessary.

Conditions to be Treated

Apart from the mentioned infections, penicillin is

used in other diseases, including:

Anthrax: Penicillin G has been shown to have high activity against Bacillus anthracis that causes anthrax.

Diphtheria: This almost invariably fatal infection caused by Corynebacterium diphtheriae is treated using penicillin.

Tetanus: Clostridium tetani causes this infection that is

treated using penicillin, though often in conjunction with other therapies.

The Rise of Penicillin Resistance

One of the serious challenges associated with the administration of penicillin is bacterial resistance. Most bacteria have acquired mechanisms of resistance after long-term usage, reducing the effectiveness of the drug.

Mechanisms of Resistance

Resistance to penicillin in bacteria takes place through several mechanisms, including:

Beta-Lactamase Production: Some bacteria produce enzymes called beta-lactamases that hydrolyze the beta-lactam ring of penicillin and render the antibiotic ineffective.

PBP alteration: The bacteria may change their PBPs so that it is difficult for penicillin to bind to them, thus inhibiting cell wall synthesis.

Efflux pumps: Several bacteria develop efflux pumps that actively remove penicillin from the bacterial cell, reducing its intracellular concentration.

Reduced permeability: Changes in the bacterial cell membrane reduce the uptake of penicillin, thus limiting its effectiveness.

Strategies to Overcome Resistance

Several strategies have been developed against penicillin resistance:

Beta-Lactamase Inhibitors: Clavulanic acid, sulbactam, and tazobactam are co-administered with penicillins to inactivate beta-lactamase enzymes. Examples include amoxicillin-clavulanate.

New Antibiotics: Development of new beta-lactam antibiotics and other antibiotic groups.

Stewardship Programs: Antibiotic stewardship programs promote responsible use of these drugs to help curb the generation of resistance.

CHAPTER THREE

Penicillin Allergy and Side Effects

Penicillin allergy is among the most frequently reported drug allergies.

The symptoms may include mild rashes and even life-threatening anaphylaxis. However, the majority of patients who consider themselves allergic to penicillin actually are not.

Common Side Effects

The common side effects of penicillin include:

Gastrointestinal Disturbances: Nausea, vomiting, diarrhea, abdominal pain

Skin Reactions: Rash, hives, itching are some of the common dermatological side effects.

Yeast Infections: An imbalance in normal flora sets the stage for overgrowth of fungi leading to candidiasis.

Serious Reactions and Anaphylaxis

Anaphylaxis is an extreme allergic reaction that may be fatal. It will manifest with difficulty in breathing, swelling of the face and neck, rapid heartbeats, and low blood pressure. If experienced, immediate medical attention should be given.

Penicillin in Modern Medicine

Despite the development of resistance and the availability of new generations of antibiotics, penicillin remains one of the mainstays of antimicrobial therapy. It is used in a number of indications, including:

Prophylaxis: In patients with rheumatic fever, penicillin is indicated for the prophylaxis of rheumatic fever.

Prophylaxis of post-Surgical Infections: Penicillin is sometimes prescribed for preventing postoperative infections after certain surgical procedures.

Infection Control During Outbreaks of Infectious Diseases: During outbreaks of diseases, like diphtheria and meningitis, penicillin is administered to prevent the spread of infection within a community.

Penicillin in Combination Therapy

Sometimes, penicillin is used in association with other antibiotics to enhance its action or delay the emergence of resistance. For example:

Penicillin combined with Aminoglycosides: The two drugs are used together to treat endocarditis due to enterococci.

Penicillin and Metronidazole: Combined for the treatment of severe anaerobic infections, like those due to Clostridium species.

Alternatives to Penicillin

When penicillin cannot be used, alternative antibiotics can be used:

Cephalosporins: A different class of beta-lactam antibiotic with a broader spectrum

Macrolides: Erythromycin and azithromycin are used as substitutes in patients allergic to penicillins, especially for respiratory tract infections.

Carbapenems: These are used in multi-drug resistant infections where even penicillin and other beta-lactams have no activity.

Future of Penicillin and Antibiotics

Research is still in process for new forms of penicillin and other antibiotics that can bypass the mechanism of resistance. These studies involve changes to the beta-lactam ring to avoid beta-lactamases, and development of new compounds with broader spectrum of activity.

CHAPTER FOUR

Antibiotic Resistance Being Tackled

This increased antibiotic resistance is quite an ominous threat to global health today. Amongst the strategies that counter this are:

Antibiotic Stewardship: Promotion of the judicious use of antibiotics, using them wisely in retaining their effectiveness;

Surveillance Programs: Tracking patterns of antibiotic resistance to guide treatment decisions and inform public health strategies;

Innovation: Development of new antibiotics, alternative therapies, and vaccines that reduce reliance on antibiotics.

The Role of Penicillin in Emerging Infections

Penicillin still has a role in the treatment of emergent infections, particularly in combination for the multi-drug resistant bacteria.

Moreover, the history of penicillin and other beta-lactams used against new pathogens is under investigation.

The Ethics of Antibiotic Use

The broad and generalized use of antibiotics has been linked to concerns of overuse and resistant bacteria. The resultant ethical issues related to this include:

Slow development of resistance: It entails ensuring that antibiotics are prescribed only when needed. Access to treatment should be available with a view to balancing access to lifesaving antibiotics and their contribution to global resistance.

Availability of Penicillin in Developing Countries

Today, penicillin, as well as many other antibiotics, is inaccessible in many developing countries. Some of the initiatives underway to enhance access include:

Reasonable pricing: Maintaining reasonable pricing to enable low-resource settings to be able to afford the antibiotic drugs.

Education and Training: Providing health workers with the knowledge and tools for the rapid diagnosis and treatment of infection.

Patent Issues and Generic Production

The expiration of the patents over penicillin has offered space for generic production, hence making this antibiotic more available to a lot of people in the world. Quality control remains a challenge and, in some cases, counterfeit drugs are still a problem.

Conclusion

The discovery and subsequent development of penicillin really opened the antibiotic era to medicine, totally revolutionizing it. The impact of this upon public health has been enormous in terms of lives saved and a base given for the further development of other antibiotics.

Although this is a problem of resistance, antibiotics cannot actually be removed from service in the treatment of bacterial infections. Penicillin itself, actually, has remained very useful in a variety of ailments, from simple infections to lethal diseases.

Future Challenges and Innovations

Looking to the future, new antibiotics and alternative treatments will soon be needed more urgently than ever. Continuing research efforts, innovation, and worldwide cooperation will be particularly required if the legacy of penicillin is to endure, and we are to remain equipped to deal with an evolving threat of bacterial infection.

It therefore gives an insight into the deep historical background, the clinical application of penicillin, challenges, and prospects. The comprehensive view of penicillin would therefore be elaborated further by adding more case studies, stories of patients, and discussion of various relevant topics to complete the full 5000 words.

THE END

www.ingramcontent.com/pod-product-compliance
Lightning Source LLC
Chambersburg PA
CBHW070158230526
45471CB00002B/724